# The Everyday Superfoods

*Enjoy a superfood diet on a budget*

## Marianne Duvall.

**ISBN:** 9781729491256

# Contents

# Introduction

Superfoods

The very word conjures up some exotic, newly discovered, difficult to get – and expensive – berries.

We have been conditioned to think that superfoods are something special.

Well they are – just not in the rare and expensive kind of way.

Superfoods are all around us.

They are fruit and veg that are full of the minerals and vitamins that we need for good health.

They are the natural source of all the goodness that we think we need to add with supplements and vitamin tablets.

But Superfoods aren't for the rich and picky, they aren't just for the famous, fastidious, fashionable folk featuring in the latest aspirational magazines.

Superfoods are for all of us and it's time that we took back the idea into our normal lives.

So I have written this book to introduce you to the everyday magic of the ordinary grocery store.

That often overlooked part of the food shop, the section that you walk straight past on your way to the processed foods on the shelves and in the freezer section.

In this book I hope to make you look again at the humble carrot and the abused cauliflower, to think again about the forgotten broccoli and the left in the dark leeks.

They all have great things to offer and they can transform your health without costing you a fortune - in fact you will be able to save money while you embrace the superfood revolution. Real food is much cheaper than processed foods and cooking will always save you money over a take-away.

# What is a Superfood?

*a nutrient-rich food considered to be especially beneficial for health and well-being*

That's the dictionary definition of a superfood, but the word has been hijacked in recent years by the marketing gurus and they have created an entire industry based on exotic and expensive products.

All 'real' foods give us some of the vitamins and minerals that we need for good health, but there are some that are more equal than others, and these are the superfoods.

What do I mean by 'real' food?

Unfortunately, many of the things that we have in our freezers, fridges and in our cupboards can hardly be classified as food at all. They are processed beyond recognition and devoid of any of the nutrients that we need from our food.

They are full of sugars, salt processed fats and trans-fatty acids and preservatives.

They are loaded with chemicals that we can't even pronounce, E numbers and colourings.

They are empty calories.

Calories that contribute to nothing but our waistline.

And it's not only the waistline that suffers.

So many of our modern illnesses are caused by lack of the right nutrients, you can even be eating yourself sick without even knowing it. Many 'healthy' snacks are loaded with empty calories and are no better for your health than a candy bar.

Even in our world of non-stop, easy food, there are many people suffering from malnutrition. Not the malnutrition caused by drought and famine, but a self-inflicted malnutrition of too much fast food but not enough real food.

It can be caused by restricting your diet too much, living on empty calories, living on highly processed foods.

It can happen to the young who are too body conscious, the elderly who don't always have access to good food or don't have much appetite, it can happen to anyone who is too busy to think about food and just grabs a takeaway or easy snack or those that think they can't afford a healthy diet.

It happens when you're not eating enough of the right food to really feed your body with the vitamins, minerals and nutrients that it needs to not only survive but thrive, both now and into the future.

The idea that we can have an epidemic of malnutrition in our rich western world is shameful and it's time we tackled it with some basic information and the truth that basic, cheap, real fruit and vegetables are the real superfoods.

So it's time to rediscover real food, and the real, everyday superfoods that can be found in any store, not just health stores or up-market grocers.

Superfoods come in all sorts of shapes, from the Vitamin C powerhouse that is a red bell pepper to the antioxidant superstar, dark chocolate. (yes, chocolate is a superfood, as long as it's dark and real chocolate)

The superfoods that I have listed in this book are everyday, real foods that punch above their weight in terms of the nutrients that they provide. They are referred to as nutrient dense. but they are easy to include in your everyday diet.

Easy in all ways.

Easy to source, easy to prepare, easy to add into your normal diet and easy to afford.

Some of them are great for vitamins, some for minerals, some for fibre and some for antioxidants but all of them will give you a boost of health giving, good nutrition without you having to resort to something exotic, difficult to find and expensive.

Some can help control blood sugar levels, some lower cholesterol naturally.

Some can help protect you against heart disease and cancers, some will help with stomach and digestive problems, others can help prevent or control diabetes and Alzheimer's and of course a good diet with plenty of fruit and vegetables will help improve anyone's health, give more energy and help with weight control.

But how do you get the best out of your superfoods?

Well, the fresher the better.

Obviously, the very best is if you can grow it yourself and grow organically and it's surprising what you can grow even in a small yard or on a balcony.

Growing your own certainly cuts down on food miles.

The next step is to try and buy fresh and in season. If you buy in season it is more likely to be grown locally and without being forced, and again that cuts down on food miles and increases the nutrient content because it has had time to develop naturally.

The vitamin and nutrient content of food starts to degrade as soon as it has been picked, so the longer it takes to get to your plate, the fewer vitamins you get.

An extra benefit of fresh and in season is that you can use a local grocery store, market or farmers market and save money as well.

Frozen is the next best thing to fresh from the field or your yard.

Produce is frozen within a few hours of being picked, so it really is fresh and it stays that way until you thaw it.

Although processed meals might be made with some everyday superfoods, many of them will have lost all their benefits in the processing and will have added ingredients such as too much salt (also labelled as sodium) too many sugars (things with -ose on the end, glucose, lactose, sucrose - you get the idea) and too many unhealthy and processed fats. These ingredients are cheap, add some taste and extend the shelf life of the product. Great for the food industry but not so great for your health.

So next time that you really fancy cauliflower cheese, do yourself a favour and make it in your kitchen with real cauliflower.

# You are what you eat.

How many times have you heard that cliché, or how many times have you said it yourself, without ever really thinking about it.

But it's true.

*You are what you eat.*

Archaeologists can tell from the bones of people who have been dead for thousands of years, what they were eating. Whether their protein came from fish or meat, whether their carb intake was fruit and veg, even where in the world they grew up.

We literally are what we eat.

On the other hand, what we eat has become totally different to the food that our ancestors ate, totally different from the food that we are designed to eat and much of it lacking in any good nutrition while being filled with empty calories which don't do anything but add to our waistlines.

It's no surprise that as our eating habits have been directed more at the supermarket, restaurant and takeaway rather than the field, the farm or the orchard, the nature of illness has changed as well.

Our health services are now crammed with people suffering from obesity, diabetes, heart disease and cancers, many of which can be linked to our diet and lifestyle.

This has happened at the same time as our dinner plates are filled with sodium, sugars, preservatives and other unpronounceable ingredients. Too much of the wrong food and not enough of the vitamins and minerals that our body requires to function properly.

Whether we like the idea or not - and many of us really do like the idea - if we want to be healthy, we have to go back to a more natural way of eating.

We have to rediscover the superfoods that nature provides for us.

Most of us put more thought into the fuel we put into the car than the fuel we put into our bodies and it's time to change that.

Greens are not something to avoid, vegetables don't have to be a mushy mess and fruit doesn't have to be smothered in sugar and cream

The superfoods are right there in front of us in the greengrocer and the supermarket.

Yes – blueberries are a delicious superfood, but so are apples. Kale might be the trendy ingredient for a healthy smoothie, but cucumbers and spinach are also power packed ingredients.

Of course, you do have to take a certain amount of care, as you do when making any serious lifestyle change.

Excess can turn almost anything into a danger – even drinking too much water too fast can have very serious health implications.

So don't suddenly gorge on strawberries – some people are allergic to them, and while fibre is great and a necessary part of a healthy diet, there is such a thing as too much! So do not overdo the broccoli!

The secret to a successful and healthy diet and lifestyle is balance.

An excess of anything, even water, can be too much and can even be dangerous.

There are plenty of everyday superfoods, which means that you have plenty of choice for adding variety as well as a good nutrient mix to your diet.

# The Everyday Superfoods

# The Superfoods

So now that you've seen that you are what you eat and how important and easy it is to transform your diet by adding more fruit and veg, you can also see that excellent health is not some secret formula.

We all understand that exercise, drinking plenty of water, getting proper rest and eating smart is the recipe for health and fitness.

And over the past few years doctors and health professionals have come to realize that good nutrition is vitally important for your overall health.

As much as 65% to 75% of your level of fitness, mentally and physically, is determined by what you eat.

This means if you eat a lot of processed foods, full of sugar, trans fats, MSG and other nutritional nightmares, you will be unhealthy. Your risk of contracting cancer, diabetes, heart disease and other possibly deadly conditions will rise proportionately.

The opposite is also true.

If you eat mostly fruits and vegetables full of vitamins and minerals, you will feel and look stronger, healthier and better because you will be feeding yourself with the nutrients that are vital to keep the body working properly, and it's always much better to get them in their natural form from food rather than adding them as supplements.

But we've also been introduced to a new idea in the last few years, the superfoods.

The term is often used to push the latest fad in the food industry and it normally comes with a high price tag, but there are certain fruit and veg that pack a punch in the nutrition charts and it's worth adding them to your diet if you want to supercharge your nutrition intake quickly.

They are the fruit and veg that surround us, there's nothing exotic or rare about them, they are easily available from any food store or green grocer

So what are the everyday superfoods?

Read on.

Marianne Duvall

# Almonds

People have tended to avoid nuts because they are high in fat, but they are high in healthy unsaturated fats which have heart-health benefits. They can help lower LDL (bad) cholesterol, raising HDL (good) cholesterol, and reducing the risk of cardiovascular disease.

So if you have avoided nuts – discover them again.

Most nuts are also high in antioxidants and are a great source of many other important vitamins and minerals as well as a source of protein, fibre and protein so they will keep you feeling satisfied for longer.

Almonds are high in biotin, vitamin E, magnesium, and manganese, which improves blood flow and calms arteries, crucial for healthy hearts. They are also a good source of fibre, protein, and calcium.

The fibre and fat combined in almonds can help control blood sugar levels and help with weight loss, making them helpful if you have or are at risk of diabetes.

They also have high amounts of antioxidants, mostly found in the brown layer of skin so if you want a really superfood use whole almonds with the skin on them to get the most benefits.

Almonds, like any nuts are higher in calories than fruit and veg because they contain fat, a ¼ cup of almonds contains about 207 calories, but they make a very satisfying snack, much healthier than a bag or potato chips or a chocolate bar.

It's easy to add a handful of almonds to your diet. As a snack, about 12 almonds are approximately 100 calories and 10grams of fat.

You can add almonds to a salad or a smoothie, as a homemade almond butter or instead of pine nuts in pesto or use them in homemade granola or muesli.

Making your own pesto's, granolas and other mixes means that you know exactly what you are eating, and you can add extra superfood portions such as blueberries, strawberries, apples and oats instead unidentified sugars.

# Apples

An apple a day keeps the doctor away – we've all heard that one.

And it's true.

Apples deliver phenolic acids, anthocyanins, phytonutrients, vitamin C and dietary fibre that combine to offer several health advantages.

They are one of nature's antioxidant providers.

Add apples to your diet and you enjoy a lower risk of contracting asthma, lung cancer and cardiovascular problems. Healthy blood sugar level regulation and anticancer benefits are also delivered.

The pectin also improves the digestive system and helps remove toxic metals from the body which makes them very useful if you live in an urban area with lots of traffic pollution.

Although they include sugar, they release it slowly, making them a good energy food and good for anyone with diabetes, and an apple is only 100 calories.

The obvious way to eat an apple is to just eat it – the perfect snacking food and it comes complete with its own wrapper.

But of course, there's a lot more to apples than that.

Apple pie, apple loaf, apple crumble, apple sauce, baked apple – the list goes on, just try not to add too much sugar to the mix and undo the benefits of the apple.

I like to use slices of apple instead of a cracker as a base for cheese, avocado or nut butter.

I also tend to put chunks of apple into most of my casseroles, curries and stews as well as some soups and of course, mixed in with salads.

Apples are so versatile as well as so good for you.

Marianne Duvall

# Avocado

This versatile food can be eaten raw, processed, cooked and included in a wide number of recipes. Though often referred to as a vegetable, the avocado is a fruit, technically a berry.

A lot of people avoid avocados because of their high fat content, but it is healthy fat, the type that can even help you lose weight and has been shown to lower cholesterol levels and boost heart health.

You can use them mashed or puréed to replace the unhealthy fat of butter in many recipes.

The antioxidants and amino acids in avocado are excellent for treating damaged dry hair and skin, sunburns and even wrinkles. This fruit is rich in vitamin K, copper, folic acid, dietary fibre, vitamin B6, vitamin C and potassium.

Most people think of avocado as guacamole or slices in a salad, but it's much more versatile than that.

As I said, they can be mashed (or smashed if you're reading a trendy recipe) and used instead of a butter or spread. Smashed avocado on toast with a poached egg makes a tasty, healthy and filling breakfast that will keep hunger pangs at bay.

Sliced or diced, it makes a great ingredient in any salad and if you add some to a smoothie it gives it a really creamy texture

Try half an avocado, about 150g (1 cup) of strawberries, about 4 tablespoons of natural yoghurt and 200ml (just under 1 cup) of semi skimmed milk to make an indulgent, creamy mix. You can add lemon or lime juice, or some honey to get the flavour you prefer.

# Banana

Bananas are one of nature's ready meals.

Just unzip the banana for a hit of natural sweetness and a creamy but firm flesh, the banana is delivered in a bright yellow jacket.

The ultimate convenience food, and for many of us, that's as far as it goes. But no matter how much you love them, there's only so many bananas you can just unzip and eat.

Of course, you can also add slices to your cereal or use bananas as the base for spreads, puddings, pies and other baked goods – such as banana bread.

And they're worth adding.

One medium banana delivers 25% of your vitamin B6 daily requirements. You also receive between 10% and 16% of biotin, copper, fibre potassium, vitamin C and manganese. Those nutrients and minerals deliver cardiovascular health and can help regulate a healthy blood pressure. Bananas also help your digestive system work properly and are known to boost athletic performance.

If you want to add some variety to your banana intake there are all sorts of delicious ways to enjoy a banana as well and unzipping it as natures convenience food.

A great way of using those that ripen a little too much is by making a banana bread or adding some to a cookie mix, you can find plenty of ideas online.

Add diced mango, sliced red pepper, thinly slice a small red onion, dice your banana and add some lime juice and you have a wonderful, Caribbean salsa, perfect to serve with fish.

# Beetroot

Beetroot, (beets) are another power packed everyday superfood.

It may have been dismissed in the past as just an ingredient to pickle, but there's so much more to beetroot than that.

It's rich in iron, copper, choline and B vitamins as well as powerful antioxidants which are very good for cleansing the liver and powerful immunity boosting ingredients.

Beets get their wonderful colour from betacyanin which is considered to be an anti-cancer agent, especially for stomach cancer.

Athletes have found that beetroot juice can help boost stamina and it has been shown to help with anaemia – a combination of the iron and antioxidants helps improve the blood and increase the uptake of oxygen.

This beautiful veg can help reduce blood pressure, improve circulation and the immune system, as well as helping the liver break down fatty acids.

The choline and B vitamins support heart health and can have an anti-diabetic effect.

And don't throw away the leaves.

Beetroot leaves are also known as chard and they are rich in protein, fibre, vitamins and minerals, in fact they are even more nutrient packed than the roots – the actual beets - and are rich in Vitamin K and beta-carotene.

The leaves can be tossed in salad or lightly steamed like spinach.

The roots can also be eaten raw, grate it and add to a salad to add some colourful crunch.

You can roast or steam beetroot, add it to a casserole or make soup, and of course you can make chutney or a beautiful red cake.

You can also juice beets, the juice is said to lower blood pressure within an hour and it's even used in some clinics as part of an anti-cancer routine.

Whatever you decide to do – take them out of the pickle jar and explore the variety of beetroot.

# Bell Peppers

Bell peppers, the sweet red, yellow and green peppers that we slice and toss in a salad are often seen as little more than decoration, but they are another everyday superfood that packs a powerful nutritional punch.

They are a great source of Vitamins C, B6 and A, one cup of raw red pepper gives you almost 3 times the minimum recommended allowance of vitamin C.

They are also a great source of fibre, potassium and folic acid as well as being a low-calorie snack – one average pepper only contains about 35 calories and about 9 grams of carbohydrates.

They are a great source of antioxidants and lycopene and all of this means that they are great for heart health, helping reduce heart attacks and strokes.

Although we are used to thinking of them as different colours, they actually ripen from green through to the red, orange and yellow that can brighten up meal time, and once they reach the red stage, they are generally considered to be the most nutritionally rich.

They can be eaten raw or cooked, they can be sliced and tossed in salads or added to sandwiches and burgers in a bun (meat or veggie).

They can be added to curries or casseroles, they are great as an ingredient for soup – one of my favourites is a mix of red pepper, sweet potato and carrot, about equal amounts of each.

They can be used as the bowl for a rice dish, stuffed peppers are delicious and look wonderful. Just fill them with the mix you want – I like rice and finely diced veg with a little feta cheese – and put them in the oven or slow cooker until tender and delicious.

Sliced and dices they can be added to omelettes, pasta dishes, a stir fry or roasted with other vegetables for a lovely Mediterranean dish.

Marianne Duvall

# Blueberries

Blueberries are known as being some of the most nutritionally complete foods in the world.

You can eat them raw or cooked, add them to your yoghurt, cereal or oatmeal, sprinkle them on your salad and use them as the basis for healthy jams and jellies.

Blueberries are constantly referred to as one of the healthiest foods in the world because they contain one of the highest antioxidant densities of all vegetables, fruits and spices.

Antioxidants combat free radicals that cause damage to your cellular structure and even your DNA. They help regulate a healthy blood sugar level, promote a healthy immune system, deliver heart healthy cardiovascular benefits and improve mental function.

Other berries such as blackberries, raspberries and strawberries also have great health boosting benefits.

There have been studies that show that eating three servings of blueberries or strawberries a week can significantly lower the risk of heart attack and mental decline.

These berries are packed full of vitamins and nutrients as well as fibre and they are delicious.

If you are used to eating them covered in sugar and cream, or made into jams, jellies and baked in tarts, do yourself a favour, in fact a flavour favour and eat them as they come. They don't need any help, they are delicious and make a wonderful snack all on their own.

# Broccoli

Another powerhouse of nutrition and one that is often left sitting on the shelf because of bad experiences with overcooked and tasteless servings.

You can eat broccoli raw, boiled, steamed, in a casserole, as part of a stir fry or made into soup – as long as it's not overcooked mush.

Broccoli is loaded with fibre and cancer fighting antioxidants, it is a good source of vitamins A, B1, B6, C and E.

It also contains calcium, iron, magnesium, phosphorus, potassium and selenium.

It is also very low in calories. One cup of broccoli provides all your daily recommended amount of Vitamin C and only 20 calories.

Broccoli can protect against cell damage and reduce the risk of cancer – especially cancer of the lungs, bladder and prostate.

It can help control blood sugar levels and improve iron levels, good for those with diabetes or anaemia.

In general, it is considered to be one of the healthiest vegetables you can eat, and you wouldn't go wrong by having it every day.

Make sure you eat it fresh to get the most out of it, but don't throw away the stem, chop it finely and add it to any soup, casserole or stir fry.

Small florets used raw are delicious in a salad but there's also a lot more you can do with the wonder vegetable than smother it is cheese sauce.

Try roasting it with pistachios and raisins as a side dish or tossing it in a stir fry. Add it to a pasta dish or curry.

I add broccoli to almost any vegetable one pot mix, and of course it makes delicious soup.

If you've stayed away from broccoli since your school dinners or unpleasant dishes in the works canteen, it's time to give it another chance.

# Carrots

These crunchy, orange veggies are more than just Bugs Bunny's favourite food.

Beta-carotene delivers cancer-fighting and cell-protecting properties.

Just 1 cup of carrots (raw) gives you a full 17 different essential nutrients, minerals and vitamins. These include vitamin A, vitamin K, fibre, potassium, vitamin C, B6, B3, B1, B2, E and biotin.

Carrots promote a healthy heart and cardiovascular system, they can help reduce blood cholesterol, regulate blood sugar levels, improve the immune system, are good for the digestive system, the respiratory system and the skin.

And of course, we can't forget the eyes, the beta-carotene, zeaxanthin and lutein help protect the eyes from ultraviolet light and help reduce the risk of macular degeneration and cataracts, although whether they help you see in the dark or how much of that belief is due to propaganda in World War II to boast about the eyesight of pilots rather than let the enemy know Britain had developed radar, is up to you to decide.

Carrots are an incredibly versatile vegetable as well as being very good for you.

You can be like Bugs Bunny and munch on them whole, you can grate them and use them raw in a salad or slice them into long chip like batons and eat them raw with a dip.

Cooked, you can use them in almost any recipe.

They make tasty soup, either alone or mixed with other ingredients. My favourite is a combination of carrots, sweet potato, red pepper and onion, sometimes I also add some cayenne pepper if I want to heat things up.

Most people think they don't like carrots because their experience of them is sliced, boiled until they are tasteless and then served almost cold – no one is going to find that tasty.

But they can be roasted, fried as chips, mashed like potatoes, made into a rosti, glazed, made into cake or bread, added to casseroles, curries, pie fillings and stews.

You could eat carrots every day and never get bored with them.

Marianne Duvall

# Cauliflower

Cauliflower is another hidden wonder, sitting unloved on the fruit and veg counter and thought of only as the ingredient for cauliflower cheese.

But throw off those old ideas.

Apart from being delicious and versatile, when treated properly, cauliflower is power packed with goodness.

One serving can provide over 70% of your recommended vitamin C intake with only 25 calories.

It is also a source of fibre, Vitamin K, B6, Folate, pantothenic acid, potassium, manganese, magnesium and phosphorus.

It contains some unique antioxidants that could help reduce inflammation in the body and protect you against cancers and heart disease

Cauliflower is an incredibly versatile vegetable which makes it very easy to add to your diet.

It's delicious and crunchy when eaten raw, the florets are perfect as a snack with a vegetable dip or hummus, you can also add some carrot and celery sticks, I also like to add raw cauliflower florets to a salad.

It's also very versatile when cooked – forget the standard overcooked cauliflower cheese.

You can steam it, roast or sauté, add it to casseroles, stir fries or soups – and don't throw away the leaves. Most of us buy a cauliflower and throw half of it away – the green part, but they are delicious.

Spray them with a little oil and grill them, throw them in the stir-fry, roast them or finely slice and add them to a casserole or soup.

Cauliflower has also become popular as a replacement for rice in dishes. Great if you are following a low-carb diet.

A cup of cauliflower has about 5 grams of carbs while a cup of rice will supply you with 45 grams.

It's easy to prepare. Simply use a food processor or a grater to create pieces resembling fine rice or couscous. It will last for about 3 days in the fridge or a couple of months in the freezer and the easiest way to cook it in in the microwave for around 3 minutes if fresh (4 minutes from frozen).

Then just use it as you would rice or couscous but with a fraction of the carbs and calories.

# Celery

Celery does not receive the respect it deserves as a healthy part of a nutritious diet.

Because of its high-water content and lack of a strong flavour, this crunchy, low-calorie vegetable is often overlooked as a healthy food. However, the under-appreciated celery delivers a huge list of impressive health benefits.

It contains calcium, manganese, copper, sodium, iron, zinc and potassium and of course, fibre as well as an impressive range of vitamins.

Antioxidants such as vitamin C, together with blood vessel and organ protecting flavonoids, help boost a healthy immune system.

Celery offers powerful anti-inflammatory properties as well. It helps regulate a healthy digestive tract and provides you with 15 essential nutrients.

It protects and improves your blood vessel walls, lowers cholesterol, protects the heart and cardiovascular system, reduces blood pressure, improves the digestive tract and reduces your risk of cancer.

Celery is also one of just a few vegetables that doesn't lose a significant amount of healthy nutrients, vitamins and minerals when it is boiled or cooked.

Most of us tend to think of celery as a crispy stick of raw salad vegetable to crunch on, either on its own or with a dip as a crudité with some carrot sticks, sliced peppers and cucumber slices.

It is delicious like that, but there's so much more you can do as well.

One of my favourite dishes is cashew nut casserole, which includes – not surprisingly – a lot of cashew nuts but also plenty of chopped celery (sliced thinly across the stalk) in a lovely rich tomato sauce flavoured with basil and served with rice.

# Cranberries

Cranberries deliver a sharp, pungent and tangy flavour and do need some help before you can eat them, they are a bit too sharp to just eat a handful fresh, but they are delicious dried or as a juice.

Cranberries are grown in bogs and then floated in water to make harvesting easy. This exposes floating cranberries to high levels of sunlight, which increases the levels of healthy phytonutrients that this super-healthy food delivers.

Eat cranberries and you will limit your chance of contracting urinary tract infections (UTIs). Rich in manganese, vitamin C, dietary fibre and vitamin E, cranberries have anti-inflammatory and anticancer properties.

They also strengthen your natural defence system and boost cardiovascular and heart health.

Experts have said that cranberries can have positive effects on blood flow and blood pressure and could be used to help those with type2 diabetes to control blood sugar levels.

Of course, it is important to choose unsweetened juice or berries, sweetened dried fruits can have a surprising amount of sugar added to them to make them sweeter.

This is another food rich in antioxidants which protects your cellular structure and DNA.

Sprinkle some on your breakfast mix or in a salad

Marianne Duvall

# Chocolate

Yes – chocolate is a superfood!

Yippee!

But before you rush off to stock up on all your favourite chocolate bars, we are talking here about real chocolate not the bars filled with sugar and all sorts of added fats.

Real, rich, dark chocolate.

High quality, dark chocolate with a high cocoa content. You need to be looking for 70 – 85% cocoa as the ingredient.

Quality dark chocolate will provide you with iron, magnesium, copper, manganese, potassium, phosphorus, zinc and selenium as well as being rich in fibre. It also contains caffeine but it's unlikely to keep you awake at night as it is in small amounts.

The real magic of dark chocolate – apart from the fact that it is delicious – that it is one of the best sources of antioxidants that you can find.

The flavanols can help improve blood flow which can help lower blood pressure and help lower the risk of heart disease.

Good news if you have or at risk of diabetes, dark chocolate has been shown to reduce insulin resistance.

And just when you thought it couldn't get any better, dark chocolate is also believed to help your brain. This is believed to be because it can help improve blood flow and therefore, the blood flow to the brain, possibly helping improve cognitive function in the elderly suffering from mental impairment.

So make sure that you choose high quality chocolate that is at least 70% cocoa content, I prefer to choose 85%, but don't eat it all in one day – or in a single sitting!

Just 10 grams a day can help protect your heart and the recommended amount is about 20 to 30 grams a day, so it's a delicious treat.

You can also make your own healthy chocolate and nut treats.

Break your chocolate into equally sized, small pieces and put most of it in a bowl in the microwave for about 30 seconds. If it hasn't melted, repeat for another 30 seconds.

Once it's melted add the rest of the chocolate and stir in. Spread it on a tray lined with greaseproof paper, cover in chopped nuts and leave overnight to set and cut into small squares as a delicious treat.

# Cucumbers

Cucumis Sativus is the scientific name for this wonder-vegetable. While the classic cucumber is recognized as long, green, and cylindrical in appearance, there are actually dozens of varieties that come in all shapes, sizes, textures and colours. The type of cucumber you are probably most familiar with is categorized as a slicing cucumber. This vegetable is in the same family as squashes and melons.

Lariciresinol, secoisolariciresinol pinoresinol just 3 polyphenol lignans found in cucumbers.

These health boosters reduce your risk of contracting heart and cardiovascular diseases and multiple types of cancer.

Cucumbers also fight inflammation and free radicals, prop up your immune system strength, and deliver vitamin K, potassium, copper, manganese, vitamin C, vitamin B1 and at least half a dozen other essential nutrients.

So it's worth adding cucumbers to your shopping list, but after you've sliced a few to add to a salad or sandwich, what do you do with them?

Well you can make the slicing a little more exotic by using your peeler to run down the length of the cucumber rather than simply slicing across. This gives you long, thin slivers which look very professional and more interesting on your salad.

Tzatziki sauce is perfect for dressing a Greek salad or as a dip for fresh sliced vegetables. It also works very well with kebabs, grilled meat or fish and it's simple to make your own.

A pot of yoghurt (8oz) a cucumber (peeled, deseeded and diced) 2 tablespoons of good olive oil, the juice of half a lemon. Put it all in a blender or food processor and zap it, adding salt and pepper to taste. Transfer it into a dish and put it in the fridge for at least an hour.

If you fancy experimenting, you can add garlic, chopped chillies, fresh mint or paprika. Try them out and see what you like – I add some to a serving of vegetable curry with naan bread.

# Eggs

It has been said that eggs are the most super of all superfoods, the healthiest food bar none.

They are packed full of nutrition.

Loaded with high quality protein, containing all 9 essential amino acids.

And they are low in calories – a large egg is about 75 calories.

Eggs used to be the food of choice for all healthy breakfast fans – *Go to work on an Egg*.

Then they became the target of the food police. Eggs raise your cholesterol, eggs can be unhealthy, avoid eggs!

Luckily, we're recovered from all that nonsense to rediscover the brilliant food that is an egg.

Experts in nutrition recommend that we should aim to eat at least one egg every day to get the most benefit from them.

They are a rich source of protein, are one of the few foods that have vitamin D and are a rich source of vitamins A, B2 and B5 B12, iron, phosphorus, selenium and choline, which can help maintain brain cell structure and therefore protect your memory.

They are also a rich source of two antioxidants, lutein and zeaxanthin, which can help protect your eyesight, reducing the risk of macular degeneration.

They can even be good for your cholesterol – contrary to the messages we used to hear. The cholesterol in eggs that was demonised for so long, can actually raise your good cholesterol.

And they are a great food if you are trying to be healthy and to lose weight. Because they are high in protein they help you to feel full for longer at the same time as giving you a nutrient packed meal.

And they are so versatile.

Boiled, poached, scrambled – maybe not fried too often. You can have them hard boiled in a sandwich or salad, make them into a really super omelette with some of the other superfood vegetables and I like to make individual frittatas in muffin cases with vegetables and then fridge or freeze them as a healthy breakfast or snack.

You can still have convenient food in your life, just as long as it's not convenience imitation food.

Marianne Duvall

# Garlic

Garlic has been known for centuries as both a food and a medicine.

As well as smelling delicious and improving the flavour of almost any food – even a humble slice of bread – this simple bulb is universally recognised for its health benefits.

It contains compounds that are antibacterial and antifungal, it's high in Vitamin B6 and C, manganese, selenium, calcium, fibre, copper and potassium.

The sulphur in garlic improves the blood vessels by stimulating the production of nitric oxide, this improves the elasticity of the vessels and helps to lower blood pressure, which can also reduce the risk of stroke. It is also used to help lower cholesterol levels.

Garlic can help strengthen the digestive system as well as strengthening the immune system. It can also help remove toxins from the body. And some research has shown that it could reduce the risk for gastric cancers.

Garlic contains some powerful antioxidants which can help protect us from the damaging effects of free radicals and are considered to help reduce the risk of dementia.

Anything that can reduce the risk of Alzheimer's is definitely worth adding to your diet.

It is also a very useful everyday booster, it has been shown to boost the immune system and is said to help protect you against colds and flu as well as being able to reduce the symptoms and length of the suffering if you do fall ill.

I have to admit that I love garlic and put it into any casserole, soup or hotpot that I'm making.

# Kale

This leafy green vegetable has over the last few years become very popular in the juicing community, so much so that you could be forgiven for thinking that making a smoothie is the only thing you can go with it.

But that's just not true.

Kale is a form of cabbage and is just as easy-going as the other foods on this list. You can eat it raw or cooked as well as in a smoothie, it still delivers incredible health benefits.

Combined with spinach as a base for a salad, you would be hard-pressed to find a healthier vegetable combo.

Kale is excellent for detoxing your digestive system. It has been linked to lowering your chances of contracting cancer of the prostate, ovaries, breast, bladder and colon. It is rich in dietary fibre, fights chronic inflammation and delivers healthy immunity system-boosting antioxidants. Just 1 cup of cooked kale provides between 20% and 1,180% of all the copper, manganese and vitamins K, A and C that you need on a daily basis.

You can use it instead of basil (nothing wrong with basil of course) to make pesto

Toast 85g (just over half cup) of pine nuts then put them, 85g (¾ cup) of Parmesan (or vegetarian alternative) 3 cloves of garlic, 85g chopped kale (1¼ cups) and 75ml (¼ cup) of extra virgin olive oil into your food processor (or mini chopper) and blitz to a paste. You can season to suit your taste. Once it's made, store it in a container and keep in the fridge for a week or freeze for up to a month.

If you love a Chinese takeaway, why not mix up some flavour of your own?

Rip open a bag of kale, heat some oil in your wok, throw in a couple of cloves of garlic and after a few seconds, add the kale and toss it around to coat in the oil.

Pour in about 100ml (just under ½ cup) of boiling water and let it cook until the kale has wilted and cooked.

Add some soy sauce, make sure that has also heated through and serve.

Kale is a lot more than a smoothie ingredient.

# Kiwi Fruit

Kiwis are another fruit packed with vitamins and minerals, in fact they are one of the most nutritionally dense fruits you can find – and they are delicious.

One medium sized kiwi will give you more than your daily requirement of vitamin C, nearly 40% of your vitamin K and plenty of other nutrients such as calcium, iron, magnesium, phosphorus, copper, potassium and fibre, but are quite low in sugar – an apple can contain three times the amount of sugar as a kiwi fruit. A medium kiwi has approximately 7 grams of sugar and 50 calories.

They are good for your digestion and for heart health.

The immune system is boosted by the high vitamin C content, which also improved skin health, improving collagen formation and improving skin repair from damage by the sun or wind.

The high levels of flavonoids and vitamins C and E can improve the health of the blood and the arteries, while the small seeds are a source of omega-3 fatty acids, all of which can help in the prevention of heart disease.

The fibre content means that Kiwis have a mildly laxative effect which can help with the digestive system and may give protection against colon cancer.

Kiwis can be very helpful for any one with diabetes. They have a low GI (glycaemic index) which means that you don't get the same, fast shot of fruit sugars that you do with some other fruits, but they are also considered to help with insulin resistance, which of course is a major cause of type 2 diabetes.

They are delicious to just scoop out with a spoon and eat, they make a delicious, healthy snack. I also like to add them to a healthy, colourful salad.

# Leeks

Leeks are part of the onion family which also includes garlic and all of which have superfood qualities.

Leeks have a milder flavour than most of the family and a very long history.

The ancient Egyptians, Romans and Greeks were all fans of this humble vegetable, and the Welsh value it so much that it became their national emblem.

Leeks are rich in vitamin A, B6, C, E and K. They also contain copper, calcium, potassium, phosphorus, iron manganese and manganese as well as omega-3 fatty acids and fibre

They have antibacterial and anti-inflammatory compounds which can protect you from infections as well as being able to improve heart and digestive health.

The flavonoids contained in leeks has been shown to help protect the blood vessels which of course helps improve heart health.

The minerals in leeks can help strengthen the bones and teeth, while the iron can help improve the blood and energy levels

They can also help protect the body from cell damage and being high in fibre, can aid the digestive process and are a natural diuretic.

They are also very low in calories and fat free, an average serving of 75g of leaks will only give you about 15 calories if boiled.

They are a very versatile vegetable, you can sauté them or add them to soups, casseroles, stews, risotto and pies.

Either slice them thinly across the vegetable or down the length into spaghetti like strips but do wash they well, soil and dirt can get inside the leaves.

# Lentils

It's really important to include pulses in a healthy diet and lentils are a very easy and tasty way to do this.

They help maintain good digestive health, lower cholesterol levels and regulate blood sugar levels.

They are also a very important source of protein for anyone following a vegetarian or vegan diet.

They are high in protein, low in fat, easy to use in soups, casseroles and salads and are very inexpensive, making them a really super superfood.

Lentils are very high in iron which means that they help improve and oxygenate the blood and aid the release of cellular energy

They are rich in complex carbohydrates which can help the body burn fat and boosts the metabolism.

They are also a very good source of fibre which can help lower cholesterol, and a source of folate and magnesium.

Although dried lentils lack 2 of the essential amino acids, if they are sprouted (a very 'super' way to have your food) they add these two amino acids and become a complete protein.

And while some other fruit and veggies can lose some of their goodness in the cooking process, it is actually easier to absorb the calcium, iron and zinc once lentils are cooked.

So having lentils in your store cupboard is a winning choice all round.

And they are not just for adding to soup.

Cold cooked lentils make a lovely tasty salad, you can toss cooked lentils in oil and roast them roast them until crispy and then add them to any dish.

Lentils add protein to any vegetable dish and work very well with mushrooms to create a filling for any pie.

Marianne Duvall

# Oatmeal

Oats can be seen as a boring but good for you bowl of breakfast porridge, but before you dismiss it, you should have a look at how good this humble grain can be for you.

Oats are packed with goodness.

Porridge or oatmeal for breakfast means that you are starting your day with a meal that is high in fibre, easy to digest, can help lower your cholesterol, control insulin levels and improve your metabolism.

Oats are a source of soluble fibre which means that they are digested slowly and keep you feeling full for longer. It also makes them easier to digest which makes a bowl of porridge very good for anyone with an upset stomach, suffering from indigestion or finding it more difficult to eat while recovering from illness.

You can add to a bowl of oatmeal by using some berries, nuts, cinnamon or honey.

But don't just keep it for breakfast.

You can eat oats raw or cooked, use oat milk as an alternative to dairy or use oat flour as a gluten free alternative in your baking.

You can make your own superfood energy bars with oats or prepare an overnight oat breakfast jar – which you can eat at any time of the day of course.

And finally, oats contain an alkaloid – gramine – which is a natural sedative and can help with depression, anxiety and insomnia without any of the unpleasant side effects that can come with meds.

So a bowl, jar or bar of oats before bed could be exactly what you need for a good nights sleep.

Marianne Duvall

# Pistachios

This lovely green nut is full of antioxidants, which of course are vital for good health, they help fight inflammation and the damage caused to cells and tissues by free radicals.

In fact, nuts in general contain some of the highest levels of antioxidants found in any food.

Pistachios also contain a healthy combination of monounsaturated and polyunsaturated fats. They are also loaded with beta-carotene, calcium, potassium, magnesium, zinc, iron, vitamin B6, thiamine, and copper.

Beta-carotene is responsible for the vivid colours in some vegetables such as carrots, sweet potato and kale as well as pistachios, and is known for its anti-ageing properties and has been found to protect against cancers.

It is a fat soluble vitamin, so normally you would add some good quality oil such as virgin olive oil to the food, but pistachios come with their own healthy fats.

Pistachios are known for their cholesterol-lowering abilities, specifically LDL (bad) cholesterol.

The healthy fats, fibre, and protein found in pistachios can help with weight control by making you feel satiated.

1/4 cup of pistachios contains about 159 calories and the fact that they come in shells – which can be a bit fiddly – means that you tend to eat fewer of them, having to work for your food slows you down. But that does give you time to enjoy each one – automatic mindful eating.

They are delicious sprinkled on a salad, added to a pesto mix or eaten as a snack.

Of course, they are also delicious as an ice-cream, but that probably doesn't count as a superfood.

Marianne Duvall

# Plums and Prunes

Plums arrive naturally in a wonderful rainbow of colours.

They can be sweet or tangy and are at their most nutritious and delicious when eaten raw.

Prunes are dried plums and are equally delicious.

Plums or prunes have a health boosting dose of Vitamin A, the B vitamins, Vitamin C, vitamin K, dietary fibre, zinc, fluoride, iron, calcium and potassium, as well as outstanding antioxidant protection due to the level of phenols in these fruits.

Your brain cells and cell membranes are composed of high levels of fat.

The antioxidants in prunes and plums protect against oxygen-based damage to those fats, and these fruits also normalize blood sugar levels, keep you "regular", lower high cholesterol levels and can promote weight loss.

Truly a superfood.

Plums are so delicious as they come that it doesn't seem necessary to cook them, but they can be made into sweet pies, cakes, chutney and jam, although you should limit the amount of processed sugars you add if you want to enjoy the health benefits.

They can also be sliced and added to a fresh salad or one of my favourites, added to slices of cheese and eaten with crispbreads.

# Pumpkin

Pumpkins will be forever linked with scary carvings and Autumn holidays, but they can do a lot more than scare you and be served up as pumpkin pie.

They are one of the winter squash family that also contains butternut squash and other versions of this colourful vegetable.

Raw pumpkin is very low in calories – of course that doesn't remain true if you add loads of sugar to your pumpkin pie.

They are high in Vitamin C, beta carotene, healthy carbohydrates, antioxidant carotenoids, lutein and zeaxanthin, while the seeds are a good source of protein, fibre, iron, magnesium, potassium, phosphorus, zinc, copper and manganese.

The complex carbohydrates make pumpkin an antioxidant and anti-inflammatory food and means it has an ability to regulate insulin.

They are high in fibre which it makes it very good for the digestive system and as protection against bowel cancer.

Many of the nutrients in the winter squashes help protect the heart and can help protect you against stroke and even lower high blood pressure.

And if you want to lose some weight before Christmas, pumpkins come along at exactly the right time.

It is very low in calories but rich in nutrients and high in fibre which means it will leave you feeling full while giving you a great dose of vitamins and minerals. While I would never promote a 'fad' diet, there are times when you want or need to reduce your weight and pumpkins can be a real diet superfood.

Marianne Duvall

# Romaine Lettuce

Romaine lettuce is as versatile as kale and spinach, and as healthy as well. The darker leaves of romaine or cos contain more nutrients than the paler varieties of lettuce.

It has high levels of folic acid, a water-soluble form of Vitamin B that been shown to boost male fertility, significantly increasing sperm counts, which explains why it was sacred to Min, the Egyptian god of male fertility.

Folate also plays a role in battling depression, so replacing kale with Romaine could help

Use 2 cups of romaine lettuce as a healthy base for a salad and your body benefits from 20 essential nutrients, minerals and vitamins. Folate (also known as vitamin B9) and vitamins K and A are found in high concentrations in romaine lettuce.

This low-calorie, nutrient-rich vegetable actually slows down the aging process of your heart. Romaine lettuce protects your blood vessels, can help lower high blood pressure, and reduces your risk for contracting heart disease.

It is also believed to help protect eye health and help reduce the risk of macular degeneration.

Although most of us think of lettuce as simply part of a salad or a sandwich, it can be used in other ways as well.

The long, crispy leaves of Romaine can be used to create a wrap if you want to avoid the carbs of a traditional wrap in your lunch.

Shredded lettuce added to your soup as a garnish adds an unusual crunch or you can use it as an ingredient in soup along with peas, garlic and shallots – you could also add some mint if you like.

Add a few lettuce leaves to your smoothie, it contains a lot of water, so you will be adding a burst of nutrients without really noticing.

Chop it finely and add it into a rice dish or grill it – use the firmer heart of the lettuce – with some vinaigrette and herbs, try rosemary, thyme or mint, either serve whole or slice and add to a warm salad.

# Spinach

Popeye's favourite vegetable is rich in vitamin C. Spinach can be eaten raw, steamed, baked, boiled, broiled and cooked just about any way you can imagine.

Spinach is also found in healthy juice recipes and delivers the most health benefits when consumed raw.

Incredibly, just 1 cup of spinach provides from 24% to 987% of 13 essential nutrients your body needs. Full of fibre, vitamin K and A, manganese, magnesium, iron, copper, vitamin B2 and B6, spinach delivers multiple health benefits. It offers amazing anti-inflammatory and anticancer properties and promotes a healthy immune system.

Spinach has a bad press because it's so often overcooked and left as a splodge of mushy green on the side of the plate. But spinach is not only extremely good for you, it's delicious when it's treated correctly.

I love eating it raw with other salad leaves in a delicious, fresh, crispy salad, topped with cherry tomatoes, cucumber chunks, blueberries, pine nuts and drizzled with a good quality salad dressing. You can add some feta cheese, olives, red onions or sliced peppers to mix things up a bit.

You can create a fast and fabulous dahl with just a 200g bag of spinach, a 400g can of chickpeas, a 160ml can of coconut cream and some pickle.

Heat the oven to 220C/200C fan/gas 7.

Drain the chickpeas but keep the liquid.

Put half into a baking tray and season as you prefer – salt, pepper or spices, - and drizzle about 2 teaspoons of oil and leave them to roast for about 15 minutes

Wilt the spinach in a pan with 1 teaspoon of oil, then add the coconut cream, the rest of the chickpeas and pickle. Mix it up well and let it simmer for 3-4 mins, squashing the chickpeas with the back of a spoon.

Add a splash of the liquid you saved if it looks dry. Sprinkle the roasted chickpeas on top and serve - you can add some naan bread if you want. Delicious, quick and healthy.

There are all sorts of recipes out there that use spinach – experiment and have fun.

# Strawberries

Strawberries will always be the taste of summer, even though we can get them in the supermarkets year-round.

They are also power packed, a very high source of antioxidants, a rich source of vitamin C, the B vitamins, manganese, folate, potassium, the flavonoids quercetin and kaempferol.

They are also a very good source of fibre, which in combination with the fructose content is believed to slow digestion and help regulate blood sugar levels

The combination of vitamin C and flavonoids help strawberries control cholesterol levels, studies have shown that they can help reduce LDL (bad) cholesterol.

If you have digestive problems and especially acid indigestion, try making a tea from fresh or dried strawberry leaves, while the fibre in the fruit can help with bowel health.

You can also eat the leaves raw or cook them

They are also very low in calories, 100g only contains about 30 calories, making them a super low calorie sweet snack as long as you don't ruin them with loads of sugar.

Just a small warning, take care of potential allergy or intolerance problems, it can lead to itching or tightness in the throat or mouth as well as burning or prickling on the lips, gums or tongue. Children are more prone than adults.

Marianne Duvall

# Sweet Potato

Although they're called potatoes these vegetables are very different to our normal potatoes and not related at all.

For a start, they count as one of your vegetable servings, which potatoes don't, so no matter how many servings of chips, roasted, boiled or mashed potatoes you have, you're not adding to your fruit and veg count.

Sweet potatoes are a root vegetable, normally orange in colour but they also come in yellow, purple and white.

Sweet potatoes are high in vitamins A, B5, B6, thiamine, niacin, riboflavin, manganese, potassium copper, pantothenic acid and dietary fibre. They are also high in carotenoids due to their orange colour

They are also a very good source of vitamin C.

One large sweet potato can provide about 70% of the recommended daily intake of this vital vitamin.

They also have fewer calories than the potatoes we're used to, although they do have more sugar – you probably guessed that from the name sweet potato!

The thing that they do have in common with the other potatoes, is that you can use them in the same ways.

You can make sweet potato fries, sweet potato chips, you can mash them and eat like that or use to top a pie.

You can include them in a chilli or a curry, make sweet potato soup or have a baked sweet potato.

They are as versatile as their namesake but much better for your health.

# Tomatoes

These beautiful red, or orange or yellow fruits (yes fruit, not vegetable) are packed full of goodness.

Beta-carotene, Vitamins C, as well as A, E and the B vitamins along with zinc, the antioxidant lycopene and salicylates, potassium, manganese, and phosphorus mean that they are a powerhouse of goodness and having them cooked makes them even more beneficial.

They can help prevent thickening of the blood, lower your risk of heart disease and stroke and some types of cancer, especially prostate cancer.

They can improve male fertility by reducing the damage to sperm count caused by free radicals.

They can also help in healing wounds. The Vitamin A keeps skin healthy and strengthens the immune system, protecting from infection, while Vitamin C is essential for tissue repair and growth, helping the skin, blood vessels as well as tendons and ligaments

Tomato paste and tomato sauce (especially organic and without added sugar) concentrates the health benefits because the mix is more intense, so you need less to get the same amount of goodness.

You can use tomatoes in so many ways that they can be a staple of almost any type of meal.

They are delicious raw as a quick snack – I love cherry and plum tomatoes and they are perfect to pick up as you pass the bowl (I never put my tomatoes in the fridge, it kills the flavour).

Larger sliced tomatoes are delicious on any type of salad.

Tomato sauce is the basis for many pasta and almost all pizza dishes, and a salsa is perfect with Mexican or Indian dishes, nachos or crudités.

Tomatoes also make an excellent base for soups and casseroles.

Bulk cooking your tomato sauces, soups and casserole bases is a perfect way to make fruit and veg meals easier. If you already have the base of your meal – the tomato sauce with its onions, garlic and herbs – it's simple to thaw it out, add some extra, fresh veggies, rice or pasta and you have a meal in minutes. So much tastier than opening a jar of sauce and you know exactly what you're eating and if you buy your tomatoes at the right time, you can save a fortune.

# Walnuts

Nuts are some of the highest providers of antioxidants, vital for helping fight inflammation and damage to tissues and cells.

They are also rich in fibre, vitamins and minerals.

Of all the nuts, walnuts are the highest in antioxidants.

They are also a rich source of alpha-linolenic acid, an omega-3 fatty acid which can help lower bad cholesterol and helps to keep your arteries healthy. This can also make them a useful snack for those who are at risk of depression as the Omega-3 oils are powerful mood boosters due to the fact they can increase the levels of serotonin.

They are also rich in plant sterols which can also help lower cholesterol levels, making them good for heart health.

They are also a very good way of reducing your risk of type 2 diabetes, studies have shown it can half the risk as well as being able to protect you from diseases of the brain and cancers.

They also contain good levels of vitamin E, fibre, protein, magnesium, copper and folate.

Of course, they are quite high in fat and calories, even if it is good fat.

A handful of shelled nuts about 5 times a week is considered to help reduce your risk of heart attack by between 15 and 50%.

The recommended amount is about 7 shelled walnuts as a serving.

You can eat them raw, sprinkle them on your breakfast oats, add to a salad or a smoothie, but do remember to reduce the amount of less healthy fats in your diet at the same time

Marianne Duvall

# Watermelon

Watermelon may be a surprising superfood but they really do have a lot of goodness in them.

They are about 95% water, so they are great thirst quenchers and a very pleasant way of staying hydrated as that water is high in minerals and has a diuretic and alkalizing effect, making it an excellent choice for days when you want to indulge in a light detox.

It's also low in calories at about 50 calories per serving although most of this does come from carbohydrates (fruit sugars)

It is an excellent source of vitamin C and A, potassium and fibre as well as lycopene which has antioxidant and cancer preventing properties as well as being able to protect you from UV rays.

It is also a good source of citrulline, an amino acid which helps the body produce arginine, another amino acid, which research has shown can help lower blood pressure levels and protect the heart.

Adding slices of delicious watermelon to your diet can also boost your immune system and your eye health thanks to the vitamin A.

The seeds are full of healthy unsaturated fats and fibre and you can either eat them along with the rest of the melon or have them dried as a satisfying snack.

The rind is also edible and contains a large percentage of the goodness of the whole fruit although we normally just throw it away. Although it might not be the easiest part to eat you can add it to smoothies, dice it into small cubes and add it to a salad or salsa or even make a jam from it. So if you want to get the very best from your superfood watermelon, don't just dump the outer skin.

Marianne Duvall

# What makes them Super?

# Why Superfoods?

The reason that these foods are Superfoods is because they pack a punch in the vitamin and mineral department.

But why does that matter?

We all talk about them, but we also have a tendency to think of vitamins and minerals as something that comes in a bottle. A selection of pills and potions that have to be taken with food, but of course it is the food that should really give us the vitamins and minerals we need.

But why do we need them at all?

## Why do we need vitamins?

I've always thought that it's important to understand the why of a subject.

If you don't understand why you should do something or why something is important, then it won't make any sense and it's much easier to ignore the message.

Maybe that's just me!

But in case it's you as well, I thought I'd give you the reason that vitamins and minerals – and therefore superfoods and good nutrition – really matter in the real world.

Vitamins are essential for health.

They help us process the carbohydrates, protein and fat in the food we eat.

They help build our cells, keep our skin healthy and protect us from free radicals and a have a host of other benefits.

The vitamin content of food is at its highest when food is fresh.

Fruits and vegetables build up the vitamin content as they mature to full ripeness and they begin to lose their goodness soon after being picked, so ideally you would go out to the vegetable garden, pick your food and eat it.

Unfortunately, that isn't possible for most people, and even when we do grow food, not many of us could hope to be self sufficient, so methods of storing and preparing food are very important.

Frozen foods are a good choice because they are normally harvested at peak freshness and then frozen, so when you take them from your freezer it is almost as good as picking them from your garden.

## There are 2 groups of vitamins.

Vitamins can be divided into two types, fat soluble and water soluble.

Our body treats them in different ways and it's important to take this into account when using them.

The fat soluble vitamins – A, D, E and K require fats for absorption and this means that they can be stored in the body and therefore can build up to possibly dangerous levels.

The water soluble vitamins – vitamin C and the B vitamins – do not store in the body, you just flush out the excess naturally.

These are the vitamins that can be destroyed in the preparation of food, as they can dissolve if too much water is used in the cooking process. So rather than boiling the vegetables, steam or stir fry them, leaving texture rather than having them soggy and lacking their nutrients – they taste better that way as well.

**Vitamin A** has an essential role in vision, especially night vision. It is also needed for bone growth, reproduction, healthy skin and for children's growth. The best natural sources of vitamin A are fish liver oils and it is very concentrated in animal liver. Other good sources are oily fish, egg yolk, butter and full fat milk.

**The "B" vitamins,** especially $B_1$, $B_2$ and $B_3$ are involved in releasing energy from the carbohydrates in the diet. The B vitamins are also involved in cell production and repair, and in maintaining a health immune system. Vitamin $B_6$, B12 and Folic acid are involved in the production of red blood cells.

The individual B vitamins have specific roles in the body.

**Vitamin $B_1$,** Thiamine helps maintain a health nervous and digestive system. Good sources are peas, spinach, beef, nuts, wholemeal bread and bran flakes

**Vitamin $B_2$** Riboflavin works effectively with iron, vitamin B6 and folic acid and is essential in maintaining healthy skin, eyes and nerves. Good sources are Cottage cheese, asparagus, eggs, fish and meat.

**Vitamin $B_3$** Niacin is essential for normal growth and healthy skin, it also helps to maintain a healthy nervous and digestive system. Good sources are oily fish, kidney beans, peanuts, and soya beans.

**Vitamin $B_5$** Pantothenic acid is needed to make glucose and fatty acids from other metabolites in our bodies. It is also used in the manufacture of steroid hormones and brain chemicals and it maintains health skin, hair and immune system. Good sources are oily fish, sweet potatoes, mushrooms, lentils, beans and yoghurt.

**Vitamin B$_6$** Pyridoxine is involved in protein and amino acid metabolism. It is needed for making red blood cells and new proteins and helps maintain a healthy immune system, which prevents us from getting ill. Good sources are potatoes, sweet potatoes, bananas, oily fish and chicken.

**Vitamin B$_{12}$** and Folic Acid are both involved with our red blood cell production in the bone marrow. They are also required for the division of cells and for making protein and DNA. Good sources are dairy products, offal, eggs and seafood.

**Vitamin C,** also known as ascorbic acid, is the least stable of the vitamins and very easily destroyed in cooking. It is essential in the formation of collagen, an important protein that strengthens bones and blood vessels, it also helps maintain good gum health. It is necessary for growth, tissue repair and healing wounds. It is an antioxidant and protects against infection by enabling white blood cells to break down bacteria and is involved in the production of red blood cells. It is also involved in the absorption of iron. Good sources are asparagus, kiwi fruit, citrus fruits, tomatoes and peppers.

**Vitamin D** helps our bodies absorb and use calcium and phosphorus, which are vital for building and maintaining strong and healthy bones. Good sources of vitamin D are dairy products (apart from low fat versions), oily fish, eggs and fortified margarine and breakfast cereals. We also produce a form of vitamin D in our skin with the help of sunlight, which is why it is important to spend some time outside in the sun, although it's not an excuse for lots of sunbathing.

**Vitamin E** is a powerful antioxidant. It prevents the oxidation of fatty acids in the cell membranes and protects our cells from damage. It also maintains healthy skin, heart and circulation, nerves, muscles and red blood cells. Good sources of vitamin E can be found in vegetable and seed oils, olive oil, oily fish, avocado, nuts, seeds, cereals, leafy green vegetables, wholemeal bread and egg yolk.

**Vitamin K** is needed for the formation of several of the proteins called "clotting factors" that regulate blood clotting. It is also needed for the formation of some proteins which are important for the maintenance of healthy bones and teeth. Good sources of vitamin K are from dark green leafy vegetables like broccoli, cabbage and spinach, potatoes, soya beans, liver, cheese and fruits. However, most of the vitamin K we need comes from the friendly bacteria, which live in our intestines.

## Minerals

Like vitamins, minerals are essential for good health. They come from rocks and metal ores and enter the food chain by being taken up from the soil as plants grow. They are only needed in the body in tiny amounts, but they are vital.

**Calcium** is the main mineral in bones and teeth. It is also involved in blood clotting, nerve signals and muscle contraction. Absorption is helped by lactose, the sugar found in dairy products, and can be reduced by compounds found in vegetables such as spinach, beetroot, celery and parsley. Good sources of calcium are dairy products, almonds and tofu.

**Magnesium** also plays a vital role in the formation of bones and teeth as well as being involved in transmitting nerve signals and causing muscle contraction. It aids in the processing of fat and protein. Good sources are whole grains, spinach, bran flakes, red meat, nuts, beans and pulses.

**Phosphorus** is present in every cell of the body, but most of it is found in the bones and teeth. It helps the body use carbohydrates and fats and in the synthesis of protein for the growth, maintenance, and repair of cells and tissues. It is also part of ATP, a molecule the body uses to store energy. Good sources are whole grains - especially oats, dairy products, red meat, poultry and seafood.

**Potassium** is a very important mineral. It has various roles in metabolism and body functions and is essential for the proper function of all cells, tissues and organs. It helps in the regulation of the acid-alkali balance. It is involved in protein synthesis from amino acids and helps the body store blood sugar in the form of glycogen, the source of energy required by all muscles in the body. Good sources are whole grains, potatoes, avocadoes, red meat, dairy produce, oranges and broad beans

**Sodium** is vital for controlling the amount of water in the body and for maintaining the normal pH of blood, transmitting nerve signals and helping in muscular contraction. It is present in all foods in varying degrees and almost all processed foods have added sodium, so it is very easy to consume too much. A high concentration of sodium can lead to swelling, high blood pressure, difficulty in breathing and heart problems.

**Sulphur** plays a key role in the manufacture of amino acids and in the conversion of carbohydrates to a form that the body can use. It occurs in insulin, the hormone that regulates levels of blood sugar. Sulphur is also involved in manufacturing connective tissue, hair, skin and nails. It occurs naturally in all foods.

**Chromium** works with insulin, helping bind it to cell receptors and allowing blood sugar to move into the cell where it is needed for energy. Good sources are potatoes, broccoli, green beans, tomatoes, apples, bananas and grapes.

**Copper** plays a key role in several body functions including the production of pigment in skin, hair and eyes, the development of healthy bones, teeth and heart. It helps process iron in the body and with the formation of red blood cells and helps protect cells from chemical damage by working as an antioxidant. Good sources are whole grains - especially barley, liver, crustaceans and nuts.

**Fluoride** is often added to tap water and is found mainly in the bones and teeth, helping increase bone density and reduce the risk of tooth decay. It can be obtained from water and any food that is prepared with water.

**Iodine** is needed for the metabolism of cells, converting food into energy. About 40% of iodine is stored in the thyroid gland and is used for the production of thyroid hormones which are required for normal body metabolism and growth. Good sources are sea food, eggs, peanuts, wholemeal bread, cheddar cheese, green peppers, milk, cream, lamb, raisins.

**Iron** is an essential mineral in all cells of the body, even though it is only needed in minute amounts. It is needed to make haemoglobin, the oxygen carrying protein found in red blood cells and myoglobin, a protein found in muscle cells. It is involved in the release of energy from glucose and fatty acids in the intestine. Good sources are red meat, offal, poultry, spinach, dried fruit, egg yolks, tuna, prawns and pulses.

**Selenium** is an antioxidant and as such can play a role in preventing cell damage from free radicals. It is vital for a healthy immune system and thyroid gland and possibly can protect against cancer. Good sources are shellfish, especially oysters, brown rice, wheat germ, wholemeal bread and Brazil nuts.

**Zinc** is essential for the breakdown of carbohydrates, protein and fats. It is needed for the immune system and plays a role in cell division, cell growth and wound healing. Zinc is also needed for the senses of smell and taste and is essential for sexual maturation, fertility and reproduction.  Good sources are oysters, dairy products, red meat, eggs, Brazil nuts, haricot beans and soya beans.

# Conclusion

So, now that you've seen how easy it can be to add more fruit and veg to your diet, how it can save you time and money as well as improving your health and how it can make meals so much more interesting and tastier – what's stopping you?

Start small – don't overwhelm yourself by trying to make too many changes at once, it will just put you off the whole idea.

So start by making soups, or a casserole or a vegetable curry.

Start by getting a cookbook or looking up recipes online or watching someone guide you on YouTube.

Keep a food journal of the way you are eating now and how much you spend.

Then repeat the journal with your new plan.

Keeping a food journal might seem just a waste of time, but it's surprising how helpful the process can be.

Marianne Duvall

Think of it as following a map on a journey. If you don't know where you start and what path you take, how would you ever know if you get to where you want to be?

You might think that you'll remember everything but it's amazing how quickly a new normal can wipe out the memory of the old normal.

So take the time to keep a food journal.

Keep a record of what you are eating and how much you are spending on your food before you start your new plan. Record it for about a week.

Don't worry about this delaying the start of the 'new you' it will take you a few days to sort out recipes, tools and plans before you start anyway.

Then keep as record as you make your changes to see how your new plan is developing.

And it will change over time.

You will become more confident in your cooking, more experimental in your choices and more versatile in how you use your new everyday superfoods.

You can also record how much you are spending and saving, and how you feel in yourself as your health improves and you rely less on pills and quick fixes.

Seeing how much your diet is improving, how much more variety you are eating and how much money you are saving will be a real boost.

Above all – enjoy yourself.

If it's a chore, if you don't enjoy the food, if it's hard work, you won't stick to it.

And it's doesn't need to be any of that.

Food should be fun, you should enjoy making it, knowing and seeing the improvements in your health and above all, you should enjoy eating it.

Welcome to your new world of everyday superfoods.

Marianne Duvall

# About the Author

Marianne Duvall's passion in life is showing people how to make it easy to live a healthier life through nutrition and fitness – making small changes in everyday life that can make big changes in health and wellbeing.

She has studied how to rebalance modern life to allow space for good nutrition and activity as part of everyday life rather than an expensive and time consuming extra.

She believes that healthy living should be how we live, part of everyday life rather than an afterthought. Something so natural that we don't even think about it, we just do it.

She has developed her ideas over the years working with those living with chronic illnesses such as M.E./CFS, fibromyalgia or diabetes, developing plans that help people live successfully with these illnesses.

Her motto is 'Live Life'

Marianne Duvall


Other books by Marianne Duvall


- How to Eat More Fruit and Veg: Improve your diet and improve your health

- Why do we Need Food? Understanding how our body uses food

- 101 Ways to Exercise without Noticing

- 101 Ways to Lose Weight without Noticing